LUCY'S LAMP

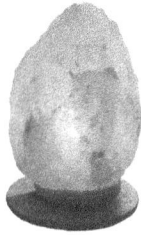

Lucy's Lamp

∽

BY
TAMMY WOOD

Lucy's Lamp
Copyright © 2017
Tammy Wood

Comments:
toceanshell333@gmail.com

ISBN: 978-1-941069-65-3

Prose Press
Pawleys Island, SC
prosencons@live.com

CHAPTERS

1
Author's Notes

When I started writing this story it was about my mother who has vascular dementia. It was about her and what she was going through. It ended up being a story about me and how I am now at peace with the disease and where she is. I often wondered how I would live with the fact that my mother was in a skilled nursing facility. I am now OK with it. I now understand that she is where she needs to be. In her own way she let me know that I didn't need to feel sorry for her.

I give you permission to take from this story. What ever touches you take it and apply it in your life. Don't let what someone said or did define who you are. Don't let accidents or sickness make you bitter or get you down. It is God's will and it will be done. Accept it with grace and kindness.

Thy Will Be Done

Memories fade into the back of my mind.
They're back there somewhere, just hard to find.

Bits and pieces sometimes come to me.
I put them together all jumbled you see.

I have no choice it is God's will.
This can't be cured by taking a pill.

Just please be patient and understand.
I am trying to do the best that I can.

Give me love and show me you care
Let me know that you are OK out there.

I worry about you more then me.
Don't carry the gilt of what has to be.

Thy kingdom come thy will be done.

These are words from God and his Son.

-Tammy Wood

Enjoy this story.
It is a gift to me from God.

2

The Years Do Go By Fast

Hi. my name is Lucy. They tell me that I am 90 years old. I have to believe them but somehow it does not seem possible. I was just washing my face yesterday and I opened my eyes and looked in the mirror. Wow I guess I am 90! The lines on my face have deepened and increased. I used to be very good looking as I remember, I still am if I wear my teeth. My teeth are long gone as they got lost with everything else of mine. I sit and try to remember things in my life that have brought me this far, something that will prove that I'm not 90. Something to prove the mirror wrong, but all I remember is this story that I am about to tell you. It's the one thing that I am really sure of.

I try my best to remember my life but as each day passes it gets harder. I do have an amazing story to tell you though. I need to hurry and get the words on paper while it is fresh in my mind. Some of you may not believe this little story, but in the end I hope that after you read it, you at least feel some sort of wonder and some peace can come into your life. I guess if I was reading this story I would have my doubt too, but yet it seems so real.

Let me start where I can remember. Ray and I had been married for quite a few years. We raised three children. They grew up and had kids of their own. We have five grandchildren. We buried three of our four parents. We worked five days a week, come home, visit, make supper, clean the house then go to sleep. We woke up day after day doing the same things.

I saw a show on TV about Himalaya salt lamps that claim to heal everything from allergies to depression. They are beautiful in the pictures and the price wasn't bad. I ordered one to put on the stand by my bed. It arrived and was just as pretty as the pictures. I lit it up and the colors were rich oranges and pinks. It had designs and swirls of packed salt. I tasted it. Yup, I stuck my tongue on it to make sure it was salt. It was. On the box it explained that this lump of salt could be as old as the earth itself. I thought about that. This rock on my stand by my bed was older then we could even imagine. Older than me now. Way older than 90. You could see the ages and different layers that had formed thru out centuries.

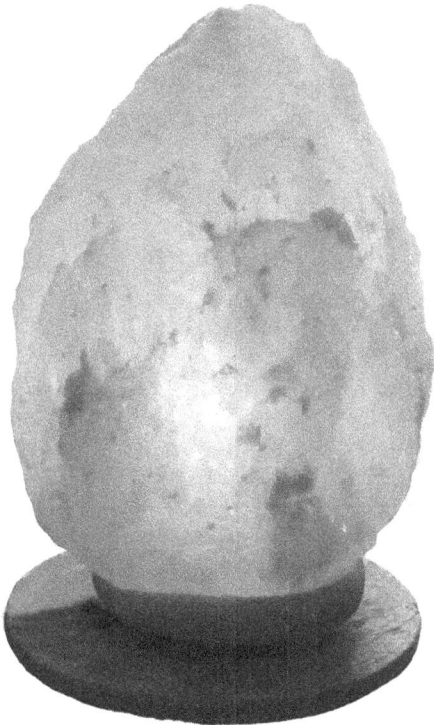

So there I lay in bed one night staring into my Himalaya salt lamp as it was lit beside my bed. I have had it for about a week now and I didn't notice any difference in my health but still loved to look at it. I suddenly notice that I see a dog in the lamp. It looks like a collie dog but I couldn't be sure. It is made out of the shape of the salt and its eyes are dots of some kind of marking in the salt. I stare more closely at it and yes, there are the eyes, the mouth and I can see the ears very plainly. I continue to stare at it. It's a friendly dog, brown, fairly large. I know he is friendly just by looking at it. I can sense it. Strange that it is so detailed in the large lump of salt.

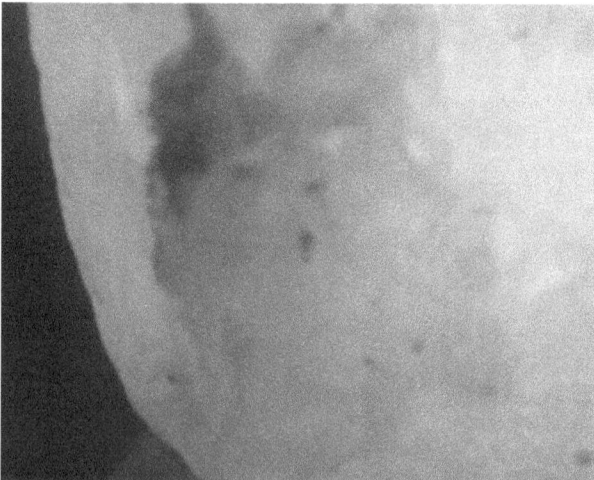

I start to look more closely into the lamp and there it is! Right opposite the collie dog is a cat! This is strange. A dog on one side and now a cat. You could even see the whiskers. It has thick grey fur and very detailed. I sensed the same feeling that she was a loving cat. This is too strange. I look around quickly at the lamp to see if it holds any more secrets. It does. I could make out other things if I used my imagination but the dog and the cat could not be denied. They were the figures that called out to me. The other things deep inside the lamp were for somebody else, not me.

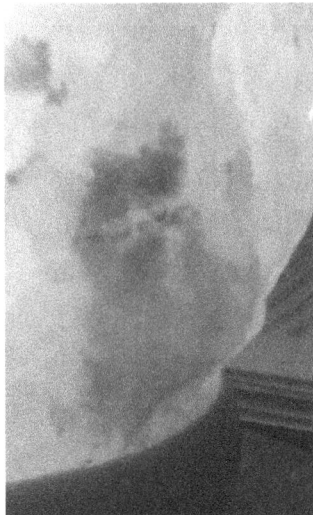

I roll over and get out of the way so that Ray can see the lamp and say, " Ray can you see my lamp from there? Can you see anything in the patterns of salt?" "Yes I see a cat", he said. "Anything else?", I asked. "and a dog", he replied rather calmly.

3

They Come To Us

I could not stop walking into the bedroom during the day to look into the lamp. It stood there lit on my night stand 24 hours a day so that it could purify the air and heal me. But it was the cat and the dog that I came to see. I named the cat Whiskers and the dog Little Guy. They were so beautifully placed in the patterns of the salt. How long have they been there? Were they designed when they carved the salt out of the earth or did they lay beneath the soil for hundreds of years waiting to be seen?

Anyway, in March my 58th birthday came and went like everything else. Ray's birthday was in June and was approaching fast. Pretty soon he would be sixty years old.

We woke up that beautiful birthday day the same way we did any other day. I looked at Ray and said, "Happy 60th Birthday!" I can't remember what he said but he was not excited nor upset. It was just another day. I turned over in bed and looked into my lamp to say good morning to Whiskers and Little Guy. To my surprise they were gone! I rubbed my eyes, hopped out of bed and picked the lamp up to have a closer look.

Where Whiskers used to be was no longer gray. It was a light pinkish color like the rest of the lamp. The eyes, nose and mouth were gone. It looked nothing at all like a cat. I looked over at where Little Guy used to be and the same thing happened. The lamp had lost its sense of wonder and I felt this tremendous sense of loss. Little Guy and Whiskers had become this little secret of mine. I loved to look at them. They were my friends. I sat on the side of the bed and tried to imagine what could have happened. The salt must of gotten too warm and changed some of the shape. I sat on the edge of the bed mourning my loss.

Ray was in the kitchen making some coffee and I heard him holler out "Lucy, come and look. We have some company." I walked out of the bedroom and around the kitchen corner and saw Ray looking out the atrium door at something. I got closer and saw it was a black and white schnauzer dog and a thick coated gray cat. The cat was definitely Whiskers. I recognized her right away. The dog looked a little different then Little Guy. I squinted my eyes and looked really hard and yes it is him. I thought by looking at the lamp that he was brown, but no that was definitely him. Those eyes. They sat outside on the porch looking in at us as if to say, "let us in."

"Ray, its Little Guy and Whiskers from the salt lamp. They came to us." I said without thinking how ridicules it sounded. Ray did not seem too surprised and to tell you the truth I was pretty calm about it too. It all seemed so natural that the dog and cat would pop out of the lamp and pay us a visit just when we needed something to happen. I think that is why we accepted it so gracefully is because we needed it. That something that just grabs you and lets you know that everything is going to be all right.

We embraced and welcomed them.

We let them in and Whiskers ran over to Ray and sat at his feet. Little Guy ran over to me and sat at my feet. It was settled. It was an understanding. Little Guy was my dog and Whiskers was Ray's cat.

Ray went to the store and picked up some small feeding bowls and some cat and dog food. We set the fresh water and food on the floor but they must not have been hungry or thirsty. They wanted nothing to do with it. Come to think of it they never really ate much. I worried about that often but when ever I mentioned it my daughter would take them to the vet and she reported back that the vet said that they were fine.

The day that they arrived Ray and I ate breakfast then went out for a walk. Little Guy running playfully chasing squirrels and Whiskers in Ray's arms. We met some neighbors and talked about the weather and the news on TV. No one asked about where or when we got these two pets. It was as if we had always had them. It was a really strange thing but I just try not to think about it. Ray seems so happy with his new companion and I just adored Little

Guy. Some times, but not often, the neighbors would bend down to pet Little Guy on the head or stroke Whiskers gray fur. They seemed to know their names too. "Hey Little Guy. How are you today?" or "Whiskers your fur is always so soft and shiny."

Ray started to get the spring back in his step and I was so happy. We started to feel the love for each other again. We laughed and played around. We had our pets and they loved us unconditionally. We had each other and it was enough. The days were filled with playful love and each day started and ended with a kiss. This was what life should be. Everyday held a new memory and purpose.

Age did not matter. I could and did grow old without a worry or second thought. Ray and I had a little secret that we never talked about. Our love for each other was real. Life had handed us a gift that we embraced with wonder, but without questions.

4
Never Grow Old

This part of our lives was the best. Little Guy and Whiskers never showed signs of age the way that Ray and I did. They were just as playful and young spirited as the day they showed up at the door. No one ever noticed or said anything about the fact that we had these two pets for over 20 years and they never grew old. I guess that Ray must have noticed but he never said anything. I noticed but like Ray I never brought it up. We were so happy the four of us.

I remember one summer day, or was it winter? I'm getting confused at all of the details. Well one day I do remember that we all went for a ride in the car and for some unknown reason Little Guy reached around from the back seat and licked Ray on the face while he was driving the car. Just as that was happening, Whiskers jumped out of Ray's lap and got into mine. This was highly unusual because Whiskers hardly ever left Ray's side and Little Guy never paid Ray any mind. We looked at each other and smiled. "We laughed all of the way home that day didn't we Little Guy?"

I'm trying to remember some of the other events that happened to us in all of those years. Yes, I remember one Christmas we had bought them both toys to put under the tree. They both woke up so playful and we were so happy and excited as we watched them open up their presents. Whiskers was very dainty as she pulled the paper away while Little Guy tore and shook the paper as it fell from the gifts. I remember that we bought Whiskers a small kitchen set and Little Guy some hand held wrestlers. It was the best Christmas.

I am sure that there are more stories of these 20 years but as I think back nothing comes to mind. I just know that we were happy and that is all that counts. Wait, 20 years with just memories of riding in the car and one day at Christmas? Something is wrong. Let me think about it.......

Oh yah, one time Ray was in the hospital and I had to sneak Whiskers in to see him. They were both excited to see each other. I can't remember how I got a cat into the hospital but I know that I did. Or maybe it was our son that I snuck in. No, it was Whiskers I'm sure of it. I can still see Ray's face when it lit up after seeing his beloved cat coming to visit him in the hospital.

Little Guy would get mad when I tried to leave the house without him. He would bite at my shoes and pull on me as if to say, "Please don't leave me."

One winter he took all of his toys outside in the snow. He would sneak them out. In the spring the snow melted to find all of these wet, decaying, stinking stuffed animals laying in pools of mud. It looked like a stuffed animal grave yard. Yuck.

Little Guy was quite a little stinker. He one time he stole Ray's hearing aids and brought them out thru the dog door and placed them on top of the snow. It was days before we found them... Oh yeah, and Ray's teeth. He took them outside too. Little Guy, what are we going to do with you?

I remember that Whiskers would sit on Ray's lap at night and Ray would ask Whiskers what he did that day. Of course Whiskers did not replay but Ray would always ask just the same. Ray would put his fingers to Whiskers mouth and pretend that he bit him. Then we would all laugh.

I used to be an antique dealer and sell antiques at flea markets. If I remember right Little Guy would stay home and Ray would watch him for me. I do remember that one day Little Guy got on my scooter and we went for a little ride in the driveway.

Such happy times. I wish that I could remember more but its harder and harder these days to remember. As I think of more I will write them down and tell them to you later.

5

Back In The Lamp

It was twenty years to the day. On Ray's 80th birthday. This memory is still very clear. I woke up to discover that Ray had passed away in the night. He laid by my side with a smile on his face as if to say that he was OK and that everything was going to be alright. The pain that I felt was unbearable. My friend, my love, my companion was gone. He left me alone in this world. How could I live in a word without him. How could he leave me here by myself. I'm alone and afraid.

Just then I was reminded that I was not alone. I heard a whine from under the covers and Little Guy popped his head out to lick my face. He was letting me know that he was never going to leave me while my spirit was still walking on this earth. I was still in shock and turned to get out of bed and call the ambulance when my eyes caught something in the lamp. It was Whiskers. She was in the very same place that she was 20 years ago. Her spirit was carried around by Ray until the day he died. Now she sits back in the lamp. Her grey fur, her dark eyes. Yes its her. She sits in the same place that I first discovered her.

I guess seeing Whiskers back in the lamp should have frightened me, but it did just the opposite. I felt a peace at that moment. I understood just what was going on. Little Guy and Whiskers were gifts from the salts of the earth. They were given to us at our time of need. They are given to us when we grow old and start feeling unwanted. They are gifts to make us feel wanted and to have something to take care of. They make us happy and most of all they love us unconditionally. There is nothing that you could do that would turn them away from loving you.

Who could give such a gift but God.

6

Lonely But OK

Its been many years since Ray died. Little Guy is still with me as I sit in my wheelchair at this skilled nursing facility. I no longer walk. I ride in this chair now because I am too weak to walk without falling. They told me that I fell and broke my hip. I don't remember doing that. Little Guy looks older now. His body has gotten a little weaker and he looks as though his legs are going to fall off. His legs are not as hard as they used to be. He can no longer stand and his movement has become so slow that you can hardly see it. I look at him and smile. His friendship to me now is more then one person deserves.

He will always be with me. It is understood that I will take care of him until the day that my heart stops beating and he goes back into the lamp. On that day I will see Ray again and he will go and see Whiskers. I wait. I wait. I'm lonely and do not know how I could do this without Little Guy.

7
The Facility

People look at me funny sometimes as I try to feed Little Guy at the table or when I sneak food out of the cafeteria and bring it back to my room to feed him. They don't understand that it is my responsibility to take care of him. I need him as much as he needs me. "Hey Little Guy" I say as he is looking up at me with those dark eyes. I smile down at him. He makes me happy. People stare at me. I don't care what they think because they don't know the secret. No one else here has a pet. I'm the only one. One of the other ladies has a baby doll that she thinks is real and I go along with it because we know of the secrets. We know the secret lives of these healing pets and dolls. I see it move the same as she does. It gives her more love then any one else left in this world.

When I first got to this place they asked me daily about who the President of the United States was and what year it is it now. I reply that I can't pronounce the President's name right now and that the year doesn't matter anymore. The fact is that I really don't know the answers. I want so much to know. I want to remember but I just can't. I know why they give me the test. They are testing my brain that doesn't work like it used to. They don't have to test it. I can tell them that its not working correctly.

They come in and they know my name, but I can never remember theirs. They take good care of me but some of the people who live here do not like the idea of me having a dog. I don't know why. I am consistently looking around for some of his poop so that I can pick it up, but I don't think that he pees or poops much. The other day I found a small round brown thing and I hid it so that they did not know that he pooped in my bed.

I love to talk to everyone. If I see someone who is hurting or looks like they could use a friend I go and talk to them. Sometimes they don't like it so I leave.

I brush Little Guy's back with my hair brush every morning. He loves it. He can't reach it like I can't reach my own back. He lies really still as the brush goes down his back. He never wants me to stop. I brush out his whiskers on his face. Some day I'm going to give him a haircut and get all of the hair out of his eyes. I do this every morning. I want them to know that I'm taking good care of him.

8

Little Guy

One time I forgot Little Guy in my room when they came to get me for therapy. I was already in the therapy room by the time that I noticed. "Oh no I forgot Little Guy." I told them. "Where is he?" they asked. "I'm not sure but he is probably looking for me. He does that when I leave him alone." One of the aids said that she would go and get him for me. She was gone for sometime when all of a sudden I hear "Look Lucy, Little Guy is at the door looking for you." I looked up and there he was at the door looking at me. He was so happy to see me and they picked him up and handed him to me. " You are such a smart little dog Little Guy. How did you ever find me?" He must have used his nose and sniffed me out. Everyone was laughing and I think that they were proud of him too. He is so smart!

One night I thought that he was dead. I was crying and the nurse came in and asked me what I was doing. "Little Guy is dead." I told her. She grabbed him from me and started to breath into his mouth. She then started pressing down on his chest. I looked at her sort of funny and said "you know that he is not real don't you?" The look on her face was that of shock. I must have said something funny because the whole room was laughing. I'm not sure what was so funny. She must of helped him because the next day he was fine. I will have to remember to thank her.

Little Guy got into a fight last night. I could hear him down the hall. There was growling and snapping of teeth. I was so frightened. Little Guy needed my help and I could not get to him. He looks OK now. No bites or scrapes on him. My daughter said that he must be a good fighter but I told her no. He can't even stand up by himself. Look at him. His legs are all bent.

When Little Guy needs a bath or if he needs to see a vet I ask my daughter to take him. She knows a place right down the road from here that takes care of these types of dogs. She is never gone long and he always comes back so clean. One time he looked a little different. His ear was hanging and I think that they were mean to him. Poor Little Guy. How could you be so mean to such a helpless animal?

Little Guy got a sweater for Christmas. I can't remember who gave it to him. It looked nice on him but I think that it was too small. He did not seem to mind it but I could not stand seeing him in that tight sweater. I know if it was on me it would be bothering me something awful. I had to pack the sweater away.

All Little Guy will eat is meat. I don't get much meat anymore so I don't have much to feed him. Its hard to take care of a dog when you can't go to the store. He needs meat. I also do not have any dishes to feed him from. I have this pretty dish with birds on it that I keep my bobby pins in. I pour milk into it and it makes a mess. Tammy brought me some small dishes and I asked her to bring small pieces of meat but she wont. She said that it will spoil and stink. I'm trying to keep him alive, don't they realize this? I need to go to the store and buy some meat.

9

Visits

Little Guy loves to look out the window. When my daughter Tammy comes to visit we bring him to the porch and put him on the back of the chair so that he can watch the cars go by. I have to laugh when I look at him. He sits so still. I sometimes feel sorry for him that he can't go outside. He would love to sit on the grass. I call to him from across the room, "Little Guy." He won't look at me because he is having too much fun looking at the cars going by the window.

One day my daughter Brenda from New York and my son Paul came to visit and we brought Little Guy out to sit on the grass. We sat at the picnic table and I drank a milk shake. He did not chase any squirrels or anything. I think that he is too old. He got a lot of dirt on his fur and I had to brush it out. I wasn't feeling very good that day and I was grumpy.

Tanya, my granddaughter, came to visit me from New York. She also went outside with me so that Little Guy could sit on the grass. I am so proud of Tanya. She works hard. She is married to Tim. Tim has a big belly and once we took a picture of him next to Linda when she was pregnant. Their bellies were the same. Poor Tim. Tanya has two sons and a daughter. Alex told me that she loved me and started crying one time when we had to say goodbye. Zachary and Dustin are hard workers. They used to plow our driveway when it snowed. They both sat with Ray when he was sick.

Linda, Eric and Grayson came from New York also to visit. Grayson is such a hansom boy. I have a calendar of Grayson. I don't put it up on my wall because I don't want to loose it. I'm so proud of Eric.

My daughter Brenda comes from New York to visit me. She tells me that she loves me every time she calls. I love her too. She lets me know what Ray Bob is up to. He sells cars. One time the nurse offered to call her so that I could talk to her but I was not in the mood, she talks too much.

Paul and Cindy come to visit me sometimes. He is my son. One time they brought Cecilia and Liberty. Liberty's hair is red, Cecilia's is curly. Paul knows a lot about the bible and I love to hear him talk to me about it. Paul and Cindy have two daughters, Karla and Nikki.

I love when Tammy brings Dale with her. I worry about him. His back hurts and he works hard. He is my hunter. When he is not with Tammy I always ask about him.

Paul came the other day and fell asleep on my bed. After he left they came in to change the sheets. I made sure that they knew that he was my son not my boyfriend.

Tammy visits me the most. Everyone here knows her. I think that they like her because they talk about her a lot. She helps me with

Little Guy. She helps me out when I can't find something or when I just need something. She has become the boss and I don't really like it but I think its OK because sometimes I'm confused.

10

Things That I Miss

I do know that I miss Ray. I miss Whiskers. I miss all of my family. I miss my home. I miss making important decisions in my life. I miss days when Ray and I would really love each other and make memories together. I miss being able to complete a sentence without forgetting what I was trying to say. I miss staying with my family but I understand that they have their own lives and I guess I can't behave. I'm not sure why. I can't remember.

I have a dog...Little Guy and I are just waiting. We are ready to go to the other side. I hold on to the only thing that will always be with me. The only thing that will be with me no matter what. Do they not see how we need each other? Will I always remember to take care of him? I hope so. More then anything in my life now I want to remember to always take care of him.....

Ray and Whiskers wait for us. This I know and I understand if you cant believe all of this but it is real to me. Little Guy is happy and that makes me happy.

I still have the lamp at my bedside and I always look to make sure that Whiskers is there. She is. She is waiting for Little Guy. I bring Little Guy over to the lamp and show him where Whiskers is and explain to him that he will never be alone. "Don't be scared Little Guy. Someone will always be with you." Truth is I am scared and I cant do anything about it. I'm scared to be alone in this place. There is always someone here. They are kind. They take care of me but its not the same. Little Guy is family. He loves me.

I keep my things packed. I am ready to go home as soon as they tell me. They say that I can use the stand by my bed but its not mine.

I keep my things packed in these hard plastic drawers that my daughter got for me. That way I'm always ready to go. We can just pick them up and away we'll go. I can't see unpacking everything only to have to pack it all up again.

When my son or my daughter visits me I am afraid that they will not return. "When are you coming back?" I ask them. They do their best. Little Guy and I miss them.

Sometimes more memories come to me and I go to write them down but by the time I find a paper the thoughts are gone. I'm tired and I sleep a lot. Little Guy crawls up to my neck and keeps me warm.

11

My Wish

I think of what will happen to Little Guy and Whiskers after I am gone and they are reunited back in the lamp. I imagine that my daughter Tammy picks up the lamp and takes it home with her. I imagine that she places it at her bedside and that Little Guy and Whiskers come out of the lamp and comfort her as she gets old and forgetful. This is what I wish for her. I want her to be able to remember me how I was when I was with Little Guy. I want her to remember how her father was when he had Whiskers by his side. Look into the lamp and remember us always. I wish her to always have someone.

This lamp brought me joy. This lamp brought me hope. This lamp brought me purpose. This lamp brought me my best friend. This is a healing lamp. We are all going to be OK because of it.

I now feel at peace and when the good lord is ready I'll be ready for him to take me. Ray is waiting.

Hold on to this lamp Tammy. What ever you do hold on to this lamp. This lamp holds two gifts from God that were given to your father and me. Someone, someday is going to need them. Let's hope that it is not you. But if it is always, no matter what, remember, try really hard to remember, I know its hard but write it down, read it daily but don't forget this one thing. YOU WERE LOVED. And that is the only thing you will need to get you thru it all.

12

Now It's My Turn

I will ma. I will hold on tight to this lamp.

Hi, my name is Tammy.

My mom is in a skilled nursing facility with vascular dementia. She has a dog that loves her and she takes care of it. His name is Little Guy. Without Little Guy my mom would have nothing to hold on to. She feeds it and takes care of it. It gives her purpose. She comes up with stories about Little Guy that get mixed up with our childhood stories. It was always Little Guy that was with her.

My father when he was sick and dying had a blanket with cats on it. He would talk to the cats and pretend that they bit him. He would ask them what they were up to. He loved that cat blanket.

My mom can still remember most of the people in her life. Sometimes its just a small memory of something that has happened. I tried to capture all of them in this story.

I was inspired to write this story when I discovered that I owned a lamp that had a dog and cat impression on it. As you see in the picture Little Guy and Whiskers are there.

I also just finished the book <u>The Snow Child</u> by Eowyn Ivey. As soon as I finished the book I put it down on my nightstand. I looked over at my lamp with the cat and the dog in it and the story just came to me. I have been wanting to write something for a long time but I needed something that I was passionate about. At this moment God gave me this story so that I could give it to you.

13

The Story After The Story

I finished writing this story and a strong urge to read it to my mother came over me. I was really nervous about it though. I had questions in my mind at how she would react. I decided that I would read it to her the next day.

I woke up at 7:30 the next morning with a text from Paulette. She is one of the nurses taking care of my mom. The text read, " Can I please call you so your Mom can talk with you? She is teary eyed." I replied that she could.

A little while later the phone rang and I hear my Mom, "Tammy? Little Guy is dead. I don't think that he is going to pull out of it this time. There is only so many times that he can do this. I feel so bad. I hurt. I can't bury him. Oh Tammy he is gone."

"Ma, Little Guy is going to be OK. He always comes back. I'm coming today and I'll bring him to the vet for you. I have something to tell you." "You do? Am I going to like it?" she replied. "I hope so Ma. I'll see you soon. I'll bring lunch." She was fine with that.

I pulled into McDonald's at 11:00 and bought her a fish fillet, french fries and a chocolate milk shake. I headed towards the nursing facility still questioning myself but determined for her to hear the story.

I entered her room to find her setting in her chair facing her bed. She was dressed in a red sweater and blue pants. Her upper teeth were in. She looked nice. I snuck up behind her and said "Hi Ma". She smiled and was happy to see me. She said she was just sitting here trying to figure out about how much longer that I would be. I looked at Little Guy. His fur was all matted and he was a mess. I told her that I would be right back and that I was taking him to the vet. I told her when I get back we will have lunch.

A short time later I returned with Little Guy and I told her that we were going to go to the porch and I wanted to read something to her. She gathered up the clean Little Guy and off we went. I was wheeling her wheelchair and holding on to lunch and my papers. My heart was pounding. I felt very nervous. What was she going to say about what I was about to read to her? Would she understand or take it as me making fun of her?

I propped Little Guy up on the back of the chair so that he could look out the window. We sat down and I laid out her lunch on the table. I then brought out my papers and showed her the picture that is on the book cover. The one of her and Little Guy. I told her that I wrote a story about her. It was part story, but did have some of her stories mixed in. I showed her the lamp and the pictures of the dog and the cat and explained to her how the story came to me.

She was really interested. I was still not sure. I start to read, "Hi, my name is Lucy." I continue reading without looking up. I stopped before the chapter, "Never Grow Old", and looked up at her. "Are you following the story

OK?" "Yes", she answered. I could tell she was very interested. If there was something she did not quite get she would stop me and ask me a question to get herself back on track.

I tried to read her face at this point. Was she mad? Was she going to like it? I could not tell. Her expression was blank.

I continued the story without incident until I came to the chapter, "Back in the Lamp". I read to her how my dad dies in the story and I read to her my words that tried to describe how she must of felt, when I lost it. I could not see out of the tears. I knew that I must go on. I took a deep breath without looking up and continued. The words were mumbled thru my weeping and she was questioning what I was saying. When I read the last line of that Chapter I saw her head go up and down agreeing with it. It reads, " Who could give such a gift but God."

Another response that I noticed was when I read about the another residence having a doll. She bobbed her head up and down in agreement and said, "My mother."

I don't know how I got thru the Chapter "Things that I miss". I was crying so hard. I was reading to my mother in my words how she must feel. How she can no longer walk without falling or how she can't remember enough to complete a sentence. I was crying so hard I could not talk, but I pushed on. When I got to the part about missing her home she again shook her head in agreement. Somehow I read on and finally read the last line of the story, "you were loved."

There I did it. I was glad that I got through the story. I'm glad that it is over.

I looked up at her and to my surprise she had no tears. It was then that I realized that she did not feel the sorrow that I felt. She picked up a french fry and put it in her mouth half way so that it stuck out. She turned away from me and wheeled herself to where Little Guy was on the back of the chair and offered him the french fry from her mouth. He did not take it. She reached over and started to pet his back. She then said in almost a whisper "Did you hear that, Little Guy? Tammy wrote a story about you and me. Our picture is going to be on the cover."

I watched in wonder. I was thinking of grabbing my phone to record this moment but I could not take my eyes off her. She turned the chair back around and wheeled over to me as she ate the french fry. She got as close as she could and she looked me straight in the eye said. "It is a beautiful story and I would not change a word of it. I love it." At that moment I felt very proud and happy that she was OK with it and then she added, "As I was listening to the story I was thinking that Tammy could not have written it because she is not that smart." I knew what she was trying to say. She was not being mean she just got her words mixed up.

I don't know why but I expected her to cry as I did. She did not shed one tear. I love it that she didn't cry. She is not feeling sorry for herself and neither should I.

14

A Gift From My Mother

Reading that story to my mother was a gift that I will hold close to my heart. Her reaction to the story and words she spoke to me were priceless.

I can't imagine a day that I would not remember my mother, but such a day is more then likely going to happen as my grandmother and my mother both had dementia. My grandmother, Memere, also had a doll to comfort her. She, like my mother, loved to feed it.

Little Guy will not go back into a salt lamp but will probably be buried with her. She would like that.

As far as the lamp it will remain on my bedside. When I look at it it will remind me of Gods gifts that come to us when we need them the most. When we are old and our minds fail us we tend to get overlooked and forgotten. This is when the most precious gifts are given. God gives his love to us in many ways. God gave my mother love in a true friend and a true companion that will never leave her.

Maybe my mom's wish will come true and Little Guy and Whiskers will one day come to visit me when I need them most.

We all love you ma.
By *Tammy Wood*

P.S. I'm going to go now and visit my mom again. I am going to stay extra long and make sure she understands that she is loved.

15
Thank You

A special thank you goes out to my husband Dale. He was always encouraging me to go further with the story.

I thank the facility where my mom is for taking such good care of her.

I thank Brenda and Drema for their proof reading skills.

I thank my mother Lucy and Little Guy. Without their friendship there would be no story to tell.

Most of all I thank God. To Him goes all of the glory.

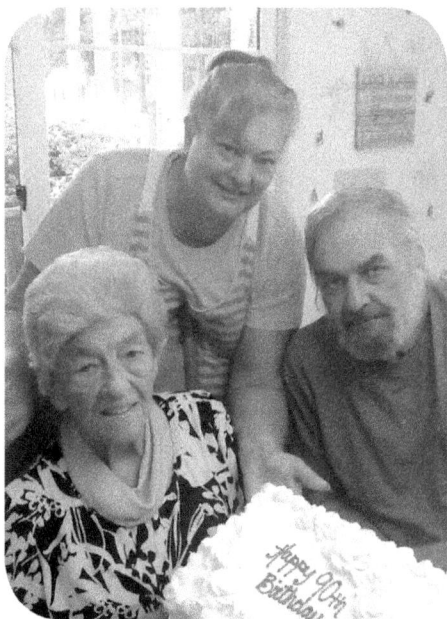

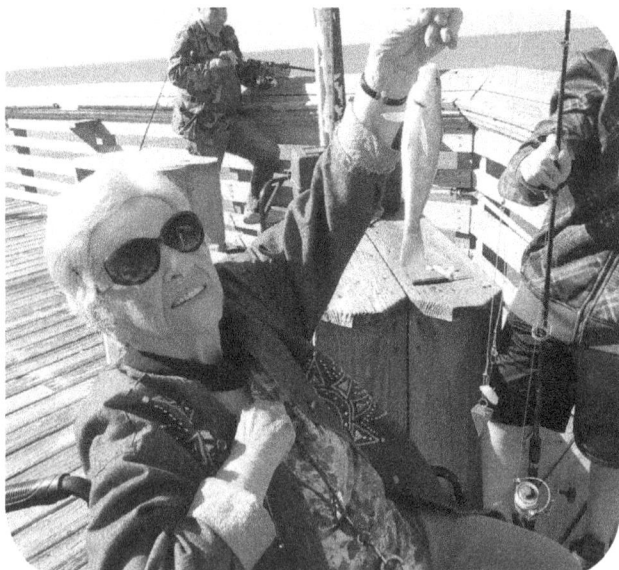

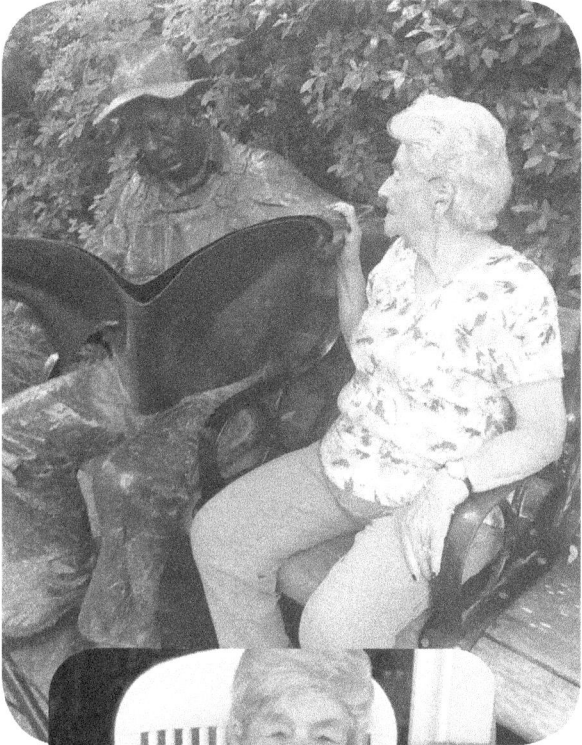

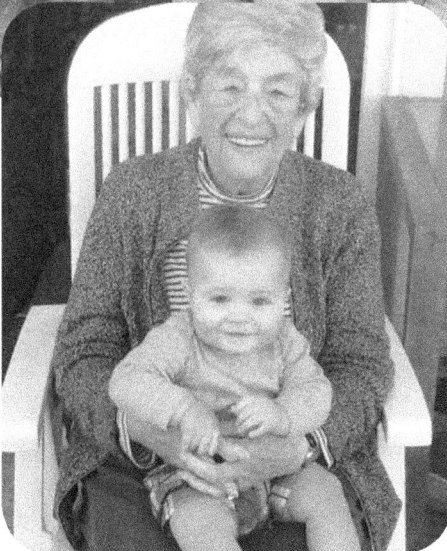

Lucy's Lamp

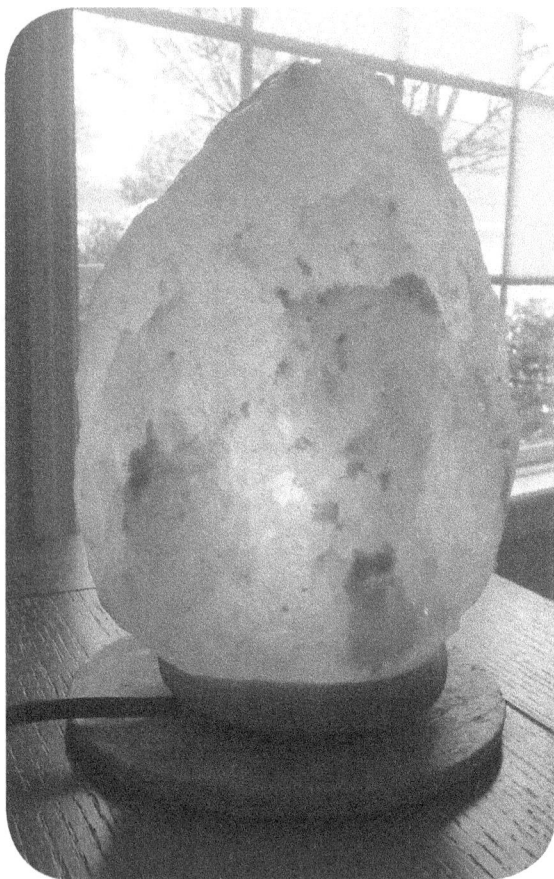

Thank You